THEORY OF SPIRITUAL CARE
FOR NURSING PRACTICE

THEORY OF SPIRITUAL CARE FOR NURSING PRACTICE

Bonnie Weaver Battey, Ph.D., R.N.

The manuscript is to be presented at the International Congress of Nurses, St. Petersburg, Russia, September 28-30, 2009. With the author's permission, it will also be published in three Russian Journals: "Scientific Investigations in Nursing", Nurse" and "Medical Nur".

This book was printed in the United States of America.

To order additional copies of this book, contact:
Xlibris Corporation
1-888-795-4274
www.Xlibris.com
Orders@Xlibris.com
62164

Contents

Foreword

For many years nursing has encouraged nurses to assess spiritual needs and provide spiritual care, a component of holistic nursing care, within the theoretical framework of nursing. However, there indeed has not been a theoretical basis for spiritual care until Dr. Battey's "Theory of Spiritual Care" was developed.

The Joint Commission on Accreditation of Healthcare Organizations (JCAHO) and American Nurses Association (ANA) have mandated spiritual assessment of all clients, yet have not proposed guidelines on how to achieve this standard. Dr. Battey's theory of spiritual care provides the guidelines for nurses to assess and administer appropriate spiritual care. It defines spiritual care while embodying the four elements of a theory (assumptions, concepts, relationships, and evaluation). It delineates how to care for a range of clients, from the religious to the atheist using the rubric "5 R's" of spiritual care (Recognizing, Responding, Recording, Reporting, and Referring) within the dimensions of the client's beliefs, values, meanings, goals, and relationships. No other work in the literature compares in the usefulness and completeness of this theory.

Dr. Battey has been my teacher, mentor, and trusted colleague for many years and I have thoroughly enjoyed assisting her, by reviewing, critiquing, and watching her initial works develop into the first Nursing Theory of Spiritual Care. Dr. Battey, congratulations on an outstanding scholarly work.

James R. Acree, MSN, PhD, CRNA

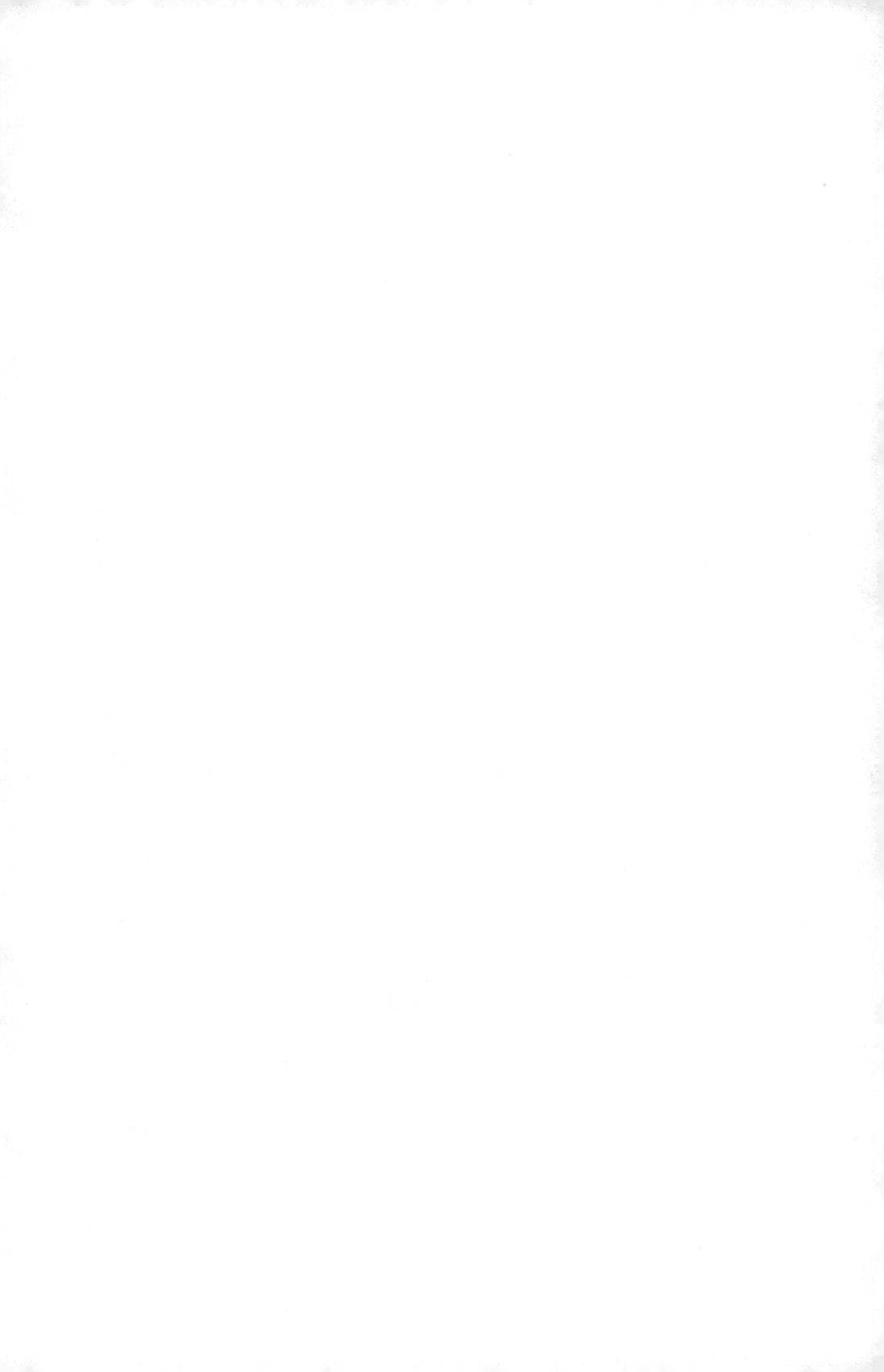

Foreword

Is it time for nursing to have a theory of spiritual care? My hunch is that Dr. Bonnie Weaver Battey, RN, Ph.D., would say, yes! The timing is not only right but way over due! In my opinion, as an ordained pastor, professional chaplain, professor and author of pastoral/spiritual care, I couldn't agree with her more.

Spiritual care and spirituality is a nebulous concept no matter how you slice it. However, once religion gets involved then there are particular practices that defines persons' spirituality, thus spiritual care becomes identified and user friendly. What if spirituality is not defined by the religiosity of a faith community? Or even if persons' beliefs is partly dependent upon their faith practices steeped in tradition, but not completely dependent upon traditional religious thought, polity, and practices, what then? What source and resources do people have to define their spirituality, thus communicate to care givers what kind or type of spiritual care is appropriate for them? These are the questions that are asked for those seeking a theory of spiritual care. Within the context of nursing these questions are crucial and timely.

Dr. Battey responds by proposing a theory of spiritual care for nursing practice. If anyone has what it takes to develop such a theory it is Dr. Battey. As a long-term registered nurse, tenured professor in nursing practice, researcher, author, and consultant of spirituality and spiritual care she has the experience, credentials, and wisdom to figure this one out. Dr. Battey begins by tapping into the varied perspectives and theories that exist about spirituality. Knowing these theories do not provide "succinct and concise direction for an ecumenical or all-inclusive, holistic perspective", she moves towards a theory of spiritual care that demands one's attention. This theory in a thumbnail sketch has four essential elements: 1) assumptions 2) concepts 3) relationships, and 4) evaluation. Within the bounds of these four elements

Dr. Battey defines not only the theory of spiritual care, but the uniqueness this theory brings to nursing.

Dr. Battey recognizes that in order to be practical about ones' spiritual care, especially in nursing practice, the "here and now" of persons' spirituality is of utmost importance. To me this does not take away the eternal significance of spirituality, but keeps spirituality grounded and "in the moment", contextually, physically, and timely. Her emphasis on the "here and now" alerts care providers to concentrate on real issues rather than things that are outside of our understanding. That being said, belief/faith, meaning, purpose, and values continue to be significant spiritual elements that form our spirituality. Spiritual formation here has more to do with how spiritual care can connect with the tangibles of our lives rather the intangibles. For an example of this, Dr. Battey uses the rubric of nursing, the "5 R's". Taking the first two, recognizing and responding, if nurses recognize well the spiritual distress of their patients and "responds in a humanizing, compassionate manner" they have begun to help patients become resilient and learn how to cope. The result is appropriate stress relieving implementations as well as relating/referring to a spiritual support systems/communities for best practices of the patients' healthcare and wellness.

Dr. Battey goes on to define and implement the theory of spiritual care through offering research support for the theory. Included in her research is the following: Cognitive Behavior Therapy, The Relaxation Response, Social Support, and Complimentary and Alterative Therapies. She also provides various usable tables and charts to define and map the unique and varied ways spiritual care can be implemented in nursing practice. But above everything else Dr. Battey has a keen awareness of how to care, communicate, and relate to her patients and clients without finding herself preoccupied with "technology, tasks, and time" issues. This comes from her own rich well of spiritual wellness and wholeness.

Rev. Dr. Paul D. Kraus, BCC, M.Div., D.Min.
Author of "Pastoral Care" (In Press) A Computer
Assisted Instruction for Nursing and Allied Health,
A.S.K. Data Systems

Preface

The purpose of this manuscript is to address the issue of establishing holistic care for nurses practicing in your hospital or similar health care agency. This requires more than just saying, "We are practicing holistic care here." Holistic care is different than the familiar bio-physio-psycho-social nursing approach to caring for people. Holism is the favored paradigm for the 21st century. It encompasses body, mind, and spirit as influenced by the environment. The body and mind aspects are the major focus of the "usual" nursing care, but spirituality is different. There are a zillion ways to define human spirituality; it is abstract, slippery and evasive—like trying to pin jello to the wall. As nurses, we are the front line soldiers of health care; nurses are the largest group of health care providers who are continually in close proximity to patients 24/7. Incorporating spirituality into one's own nursing practice or for the entire nursing staff at your agency is probably a most pressing and intangible task facing nursing today.

The hospital accrediting agency as well from the various health care professional statements of standards and ethics have new criteria and expectations for nurses to provide spiritual care. While it may be sufficient to leave the defining of spiritual care and practice to individual nurses, it is better to address this significant issue as a group through the establishment of education, policies, guidelines, and interdisciplinary support and networking. Coordination of efforts and teamwork among nursing staff can improve quality of care and provide a "paper trail" for accreditation reviewers.

In this manuscript, The Theory of Spiritual Care for Nursing is offered to provide guidance and structure to this effort. It is proposed that the scope of spiritual care needs to be limited for nursing. We are not chaplains; we need to know when we have done enough. This theory is research-based, drawing on theories, supporting research, and the study of spirituality in healing from numerous disciplines. A plan is offered for implementing the Theory of Spiritual Care for Nursing that gives guidance for those unplanned, "here and now" nurse-client encounters. Such encounters provide opportunities for making interpersonal connections that are the compassionate, rewarding dimension of nursing practice.

This is *not* to be considered *the* final answer, but I hope to provide one perspective which may serve as a basis for developing a plan most appropriate to your agency. Like clients, nurses also have so many religions and belief systems. Like a choir, we need to be harmonious, singing from the "same page." It is proposed that the computer assisted instruction (CAI) program, Spirituality in Nursing Practice, serve as a "same page" orientation to spirituality. This, with additional local educational presentations, can serve as another "same page."

Those accreditation criteria and statements of standards are so broad in scope and vague. Having specific decisions and action plans in addressing spirituality in client care will probably be helpful to all in developing holistic care within your agency.

Bonnie Weaver Battey, Ph.D., R.N.

Acknowledgements

There are dozens of my friends and colleagues who have so graciously and often unknowingly influenced the development of this Nursing Theory of Spiritual Care. It was during their many presentations, questions, discussions and personal communications that they contributed to the initiation, development and substance of this theory. This book represents my sincere thank you.

A special acknowledgement of the following individuals who peer reviewed the manuscript:

To: James R. Acree, BSN, BSNA, MS, MSN, PhD, CRNA.

To: Rev. Michael A. Jeffrey, Evangelical Lutheran Church in America (ELCA) Minister.

To: Dr. Paul D. Kraus, D.Min.
      Author of "Pastoral Care" (In Press) Computer Assisted Instruction for Nursing and Allied Health, A.S.K. Data Systems (Fall 2008)
      Instructor and Partnership Coordinator of the Texas-Mexico Pastoral Care & Counseling Conferences sponsored by Hospital Mexico Americano, Guadalajara, Jalisco, Mexico

To Rev. Jerry L. Schmalenberger, BA, M-Div, D-Min, D.D.
      Retired President, Pacific Lutheran Theological Seminary, Berkeley, CA.
      ELCA Global Mission Volunteer
      Affiliate faculty, LTS, Hong Kong
      Affiliate faculty, STT-HKBP, Sumatra, Indonesia

Lecturer, Balige Deaconess School, Sumatra, Indonesia
Affiliate Faculty, Abdi Sabda Seminary, Medan, Sumatra

A special note of appreciation is most appropriate to two people introduced me to the chaplaincy role and mentored me through 4 years of service as a volunteer "layman" chaplain. First is the Director of Pastoral Care, Chaplain J. Vincent Guss Jr., D.Min(c), an ordained Lutheran minister, and a Board Certified Chaplain through the Association of Professional Chaplains. Second is Kathy A. Garrison MAR, Director, Art of Pastoral Care, Pastoral Counseling of Northern Virginia, a Lutheran Deaconess, and a Diaconal Minister of the ELCA. (She is a former Registered Nurse).

The research and many conferences presented by Dr. Herbert Benson and his associates at The Benson-Henry Institute of the Massachusetts General Hospital and Harvard University School of Medicine in Boston have been a significant influence on the development of this theory.

And finally, to the many who are not mentioned here, that does not diminish the importance of their contributions or my feelings of gratitude for their work.

Bonnie Weaver Battey

Introduction

Implementing spiritual care in nursing practice is probably one of the most pressing and abstract issues facing nurses today. In the United States, accreditation criteria of the Joint Commission on Accreditation of Healthcare Organizations (2005) require spiritual assessment; professional standards and codes of the American Nurses' Association (2005) and the North American Nursing Diagnosis Association (NANDA) Manuals of Nursing Diagnosis (2008) advocate for spiritual care. Florence Nightingale believed spiritual care to be essential to healing (Nightingale 1959; O'Brien, 1999; Macrae, 1995).

In this paper, some perspectives of note that support this theory found in the nursing literature and are summarized. Second, the need for a theory of spirituality is documented, and the essential elements of a theory are described. Third, the uniqueness of spirituality in nursing is addressed. Fourth, a theory of spirituality specifically for nursing is proposed and essential elements presented. Fifth, research findings supporting the interventions which improve clients' spirituality are identified. Finally, application of this theory of spirituality and its use in developing spiritual care maps are suggested for educational programs. Implementation of spiritual care in a health care agency is also described.

Nursing Literature

Views about spirituality vary widely. For example, Lemmer (2002) conducted a survey of United States baccalaureate nursing programs to learn what is taught about spirituality. Spirituality is not well defined in the nursing literature and consequently it is ambiguous in meaning. Nursing faculty reported that it is included in the curriculum, but few had functional definitions of spirituality or spiritual care. Some nursing faculties teach it, but many admitted not knowing what to teach. There is even a debate developing about whether or not to teach spirituality in nursing programs (McSherry and Ross, 2002; McSherry and Cash. 2004: See also McSherry, 2006). Meyer (2003) questions how well nurse educators are preparing students to provide spiritual care. Only two contemporary theorists specifically address spirituality as a major concept; Betty Neuman's Systems Model (1989) and Madeleine Leininger's Transcultural Nursing (1978).

In a review of nursing textbooks (McEwen, 2004), many definitions of *spirituality* were found, but few definitions of *spiritual care*. Pages devoted to spiritual issues ranged from 0% for most to 13%. Only two texts were exceptions. Carson (2000) integrated spiritual care throughout her psychiatric text. Hitchcock, et al, (2003) had a chapter in their community nursing text. A third noteworthy exception is the in-depth presentation of spirituality in the chapter by Berman in Kozier & Erb's Fundamentals of Nursing text (Berman, Snyder, Kozier, & Erb, 2007, 8th Ed.).

There are numerous texts about spiritual care in health care from a religious, particularly Christian, perspective by both nurses and non-nurses. Examples of these include books by Koenig (2002), Carson and Koenig (2004), Taylor (2002), Barnum (2003), and Shea (2000). Numerous textbooks are about faith based community nursing or parish nursing (Battey, 2005). However, none known to this author provide succinct and concise direction for an ecumenical or all-inclusive, holistic perspective for the nursing staff of a hospital or similar agency; this is the goal of this current book.

Beliefs about spirituality range from a firm religious theological position, to the atheist and agnostic, to those who do not even recognize human spirituality. To have an in-depth knowledge of spiritual religious belief systems is outside the range of the nursing role and competencies. Yet, somehow, nurses are to provide spiritual care to every client. How can this be accomplished? A potential solution is to establish a nursing theory of spiritual care to provide direction and structure for an ecumenical and ethical practice.

Theory

A theory has four essential elements: i.e., assumptions, concepts, relationships, and evaluation. These are analogous to a theatrical performance. The *assumptions* describe the important aspects of the environment, similar to the stage back-drop, props, and other scenery for a play. Classified according to source, assumptions are accepted as true without testing through research; they provide a static, unchanging backdrop for the theory. The topics included in assumptions can be anything, but to be a nursing theory, four concepts are necessary; man, health, environment, and nursing. See Table 1, page 26, for the list of assumptions for the proposed theory of spiritual care.

A *concept* is a word or term used to classify or describe a phenomenon just as the characters or actors of a play are described in the script. A conceptual definition is to be timeless, impersonal and abstract, ready to be used in research or applied to a real-life situation. See Table 2, page 28, for the list of concepts for the proposed theory of spiritual care.

The *relationship statements* of the theory describe the way concepts interact, just as the script of a play describe interactions among the actors, what they do and say. Unlike static assumptions, the relationship statements are active, showing movement and change. Describing the logical or natural association between two or more concepts within the assumptions, relationship statements provide meaning, promote understanding, and hopefully predict outcomes for guides to action. Stated as logical principles and/or mathematical equations, relationships statements are easily converted to research questions and hypothesis. See Table 3, page 32, for the list of relationship statements for the proposed theory of spiritual care.

The *evaluation* of a theory is primarily based on testing of the relationship statements through research, both quantitative and qualitative. In the theater, the audience's response to the play is the evaluation, i.e., the applause, the length of the "run" of the play, and critics' reviews. In addition to research, other criteria some may use to evaluate a theory include parsimony, scope and limitations, applicability, generalizability, and importance to the discipline. The degree of agreement with known data and life experiences are other modes of evaluation. The function of research is to rate the degree of significance of the findings and to give directions for revision of the theoretical statements. See Table 4, page 33, for the evaluation of the proposed theory of spiritual care.

Uniqueness of Nursing Theory

Nursing as a discipline addresses spirituality in the context and scope of holistic health care rather than the broader sense, as in theology and religion. These and other disciplines address spirituality from the perspective of health and wellness as well as illness. The purpose of nursing is to intervene to support, maintain, and augment the client's state of compromised holistic health. The outcome of spiritual care is to increase the client's ability to maintain "resiliency" and cope with "critical life situations."

The philosophical basis of this theory of spiritual care is existentialism, which focuses on the "here and now" of the moment and the sense of disorientation and confusion in an apparent meaningless world. Existential philosophy emphasizes the individual as a self determining agent responsible for one's own choices, and it serves as the basis of other theories used in nursing. For example, Buber's "I-Thou" (1970) distinguishes between communicating with an "object" or "I-It" vs. a "person" or "I-Thou." Other existential nursing theories include Patterson and Zderad's "being with" (1976) and Battey's "communing" (1985, 2005, 2009). The potential impact of spiritual care provided by nurses is based on two factors. First, nurses are the largest health care professional group. Second, they practice in close proximity to clients, typically on a 24 hour/7 day basis. See Figure 1, The Half-Circle Organizational Chart, page 25. The "in the moment" interactions with clients often are typically brief, unplanned, and spontaneous, hence the existentialistic perspective.

Nurses are not chaplains; they don't have the healing tools of chaplains. Christian chaplains, for example, have tools for healing which include the power of prayer, forgiveness of sins, removal of guilt, unconditional love of God and others, peace for stressed personalities, the sacraments, and ultimately the hope of eternal life. Christians speak of the "real presence" of Christ at communion and in the hospital room when the laying on of hands and prayer is offered. (Schmalenberger, 2009).

The nursing goal of spiritual care is to provide an environment to support the client's development of resiliency, optimism, helpfulness, and social bonding. The role of nurses needs to focus on the rubric, the "5 R's" of spiritual care.

1. **Recognizing** spiritual distress and aspects of the client's personal definition of spirituality.
2. **Responding** in a humanizing, compassionate manner.
3. **Recording** according to ethical and legal guidelines and agency policies.
4. **Reporting** on a "need to know" basis to appropriate health care providers.
5. **Referring** to an appropriate spiritual advisor, such as a priest, rabbi, imam, or others. (Battey, 2008)

Since nurses are not chaplains, it is proposed that *nurses be responsible for only these five dimensions of spirituality of the individual client's definition: Beliefs, Values, Meanings, Goals, and Relationships i.e. BVMGR* (Battey, 2008,

2009). Some nurses may choose to do more than the 5 R's and the BVMGR, particularly when clients are members of their own faith community or advocates of similar spiritual beliefs. However, for most nurses, when the 5 R's have been accomplished, the nurses have done enough.

Many rubrics are available in the literature to guide the health providers in conducting the spiritual assessment. The rubric BVMGR is proposed as sufficient and appropriate for nursing. Generally, the mandated spiritual assessment is to determine the answers to the following questions:

1. How spirituality/religion influences this person's health care?
2. How beliefs about spirituality/religion can help this person cope with illness and stress?
3. What spiritual needs can be identified and addressed?
4. Is a referral needed to a chaplain, priest, or other spiritual advisor?
5. What is the scope and limitations of support systems for this patient?

Responses to one or more of these questions may serve as a basis for developing an individualized spiritual care plan or map. See Table 5, page 35, for a suggested format.

Normally, the nurse has two tasks: 1) to explore the client's perception of the world; and 2) to be aware of one's own personal theory of the world and how it impacts the relationship with the client. In therapeutic communication, the nurse is to challenge those aspects of the client's personal theory that seem to produce problems. Progression toward health is evidenced by the degree of change in the client's personal theory and the degree to which the client accepts responsibility for the outcomes of his/her own actions. (Battey, 2008).

However, for spiritual care, the nurse had a third task; to *avoid challenging* the client's definition of spirituality, the BVMGR, but to be aware how this personal definition of spirituality potentially impacts with the client's health status and care. Spiritual care is *relational*. What and how a nurse is *thinking* and *behaving* needs to be perceived by the patient as humanizing and compassionate in order for the patient to develop trust of the nurse and to self disclose concerns related to the BVMGR.

Nurses' behavior needs to be unique in that this is one human being interacting with another person. We all are subject to an occasional criticism, one-up-man-ship, humiliation, and the like. We who are healthy deal with it. Even health people, including nurses, need spiritual care. The research reported by Dr. Linda Aiken and her colleagues at the University of Pennsylvania (Aiken, et al, 1994, 2001, 2002, 2004) as well as Dr. Peter

Buerhaus and his colleagues at Vanderbilt University (2001, 2002abc, 2003, 2004, 2005) have identified ineffective communication as an issue of concern not only in the recruitment attracting students into nursing schools but also in maintenance of an attractive workplace for nurses. There is some evidence that the mortality of patients varies with the quality of communication occurring between nurses and doctors. Spiritual care is RELATIONAL.

But a client who is experiencing a critical life situation is special. This person requires the establishment of a "reparative healing environment" as proposed by Florence Nightingale (1859) that includes a communicative atmosphere or ambiance supportive of the relational, the "communing" of spiritual care. Progression toward health is typically evidenced by the degree of change in the client's demeanor, attitude, or bearing. He or she becomes more peaceful, calm, and maybe even serene. (Battey, in press, Lesson 6; Duldt, 1996.)

New Concepts

There are new labels for stress and homeostasis. Hans Selye's (1973) classic research on stress and homeostasis provided definitions of the cycle of human stress responses. Using the holistic paradigm, research by Sterling and Eyer (1988) and by McEwen (1998, 1999a) introduced the concept of "allostasis," meaning "maintaining stability (homeostasis) through change" "Allostasis load" refers to the wear and tear one's body experiences from going through many cycles of allostasis stress responses, repeatedly turning the system on and off. Allostasis load disorders, then, are the range of illnesses associated with the dysfunction of the allostatic system. (Nielsen, Seaman & Hahn, 2007)

> "'Stress and allostatic loading' contributes to the onset or exacerbation of many disabling diseases with high morbidity and mortality. Examples include hypertension, arthrosclerosis, coronary artery disease (IHD, MI, SCD[1]), cardiomyopathy and heart failure, metabolic syndrome and insulin resistant diabetes, autoimmune diseases, and possibly HIV/AIDS?[2], Alzheimer's?, anxiety and depression." (Fricchione, 2004)

---

[1] IHD or ischemic heart disease; MI or myocardial infarction; and SCD or sudden cardiac death.

[2] The question marks are to indicate that the research findings only suggest these are included.

This concept of allostatic load has become a benchmark for a cumulative measure of physiological dis-regulation over multiple body systems.

Research Support for Theory

Researchers have pooled physiological measures from the new technology, i.e., scans, screenings, and testing, to determine if there could be a predictor of disease and deterioration of the human system. Ten physiological measures or "markers" of spiritual distress were identified. See Table 2, Concepts, page 31, #13 for the list of markers. In reviewing patients' history and physical assessment, these markers need to be recognized not only as physiological concerns but also as signs of spiritual distress.

There is strong research evidence of the effectiveness of four interventions for spiritual distress. See Table 4, Evaluation, page 33, #1, Relevant Research.

Cognitive Behavior Therapy. The old view of *either* cognitive *or* behavioral theoretical approach to therapy now has a new approach: *both* cognitive *and* behavioral. Cognitive Behavioral Therapy (CBT) has to do with changing the patient's belief/disbelief system in a therapeutic manner. This is *not* attempting to change the person's belief/disbelief system regarding the existence of a higher being or God or religious beliefs. It has been used very successfully in cases of anxiety, depression, and chronic pain, according to Dr. Fricchione (2004). The person is taught how to substitute positive thoughts for negative, automatic thoughts. For example, Seligman, et al. (1999) studied college students at risk for anxiety and depression over a three year period. As a treatment intervention, he gave them cognitive behavior therapy and stress management. Findings show a reduction in moderate to severe depression and anxiety over a three year period. This is an example of a mind/body intervention preventing an illness through stress buffering. (Fricchione, 2004). Other studies of spiritual distress include those by Enright (2001) and Flanigan (1992). Research related to Cognitive Behavioral therapy is also available at the National Institute of Health (2006) in the United States.

The Relaxation Response. Herbert Benson, M.D. (1975) is the earliest Western investigator of the effects of meditation on health. As the primary investigator of the Relaxation Response (RR), Dr. Benson (1974, 2004) teaches that self-induced stimulus can give one a lot of power in breaking allostatic loadings and developing stress buffering by breaking the train of individual thoughts. Basically RR is prayer and/or meditation. Investigators include Matthews (1999) and Dossey (1993), among others.

Social Support. Social support is having family and friends, neighbors and co-workers with whom to talk about concerns, often obtaining good advice, in an accepting interpersonal climate. Both the number of supporters and the quality of the relationships contribute to stress buffering. Social distress is associated with poor health, and it follows a pattern. First, this involves an individual's appraisal of the demands and the capacity of adaptive abilities. Next, the person decides what is going to be too stressful. Lack of social support or not enough of it can affect one's health negatively. Examples of deficient social support include isolation typically associated with illness, as well as other factors, such as family discord, job related issues, retirement, race and other social bias, and many others. The Thomas Holmes and Richard Rahe (1971) "Social Readjustment Rating Scale" is a benchmark tool for research and screening of social stressors with specific codification. Other investigators include Beckman and Syme (1979) and Levin (2001).

Complimentary and Alternative Therapies. The National Institute for Complimentary and Alternative Medicine is the lead agency in the United States for scientific research on the diverse medical and health care systems, practices, and herbal products that are not generally considered part of conventional medicine. Many of these therapies provide remarkable interventions for stress buffering and counteracting spiritual distress. Some are commonly included as a part of nursing practice, such as therapeutic or healing touch, herbal therapy, aroma therapy, music therapy, and many others.

Implementation of Spiritual Care Theory

Too often we have a preoccupation with technology, tasks, and time rather than caring, communication, and clients. Awareness of the spiritual dimensions of humans is often pushed aside. However, it is that spiritual dimension that lies at the core of nursing. The demands of keeping up with the scientific breakthroughs, contamination precautions, insurance restrictions to supplies or hospital days, emergencies, and duty schedules place incredible pressure on nursing staff and other health care professionals. Yet it is the nurses who provide a research based and significant intervention by just "being there"—the *social support* in augmenting clients' resilience and coping.

Implementing spiritual care in your agency and supporting individual nurses' efforts can be accomplished by forming a task team to develop guidelines, educational programs, and administrative policies. **In**

preparation for their work, the task team members may be asked to participate in an educational program such as the computer assisted instruction (CAI), Spirituality in Nursing Practice (Battey, in press). This program provides not only case studies and stories but also a research based, organized, and focused approach to incorporating spiritual care in the practice of individual nurses.

Within the educational program, a Spiritual Care Map may be used by the participants in analyzing client case situations. See Table 5, page 35, for a sample care map. A sample case situation may be provided for consideration. See Table 6, page 36, for a sample case description of a woman with ovarian cancer (Battey, in press). A key consideration in this case is to provide a way for the women to be an influence on her children's lives after her death. Suggestions include journaling, recording, or video taping whatever it is she wants to say to them. Relatives may assume responsibility for making these available to her children on their graduation, marriage, etc. Similar case studies can be developed based on the client population served by your agency.

Perhaps an educational program similar to the computer assisted instruction, Spirituality in Nursing Practice (Battey, in press; see back cover) for the nursing staff might be arranged by other resources. Whatever tactic is used, the approach needs to be ecumenical because of the wide variety of beliefs. It may be a Jewish hospital, a Christian or Buddhist nurse, caring for an Atheist, Mormon, Islamic, or Hindu patient. The nurses cannot be expected to know about each one of these belief systems, but need to learn what question to ask and to listen for the individual's client's spiritual definition that may impact on the patient's health care.

In many hospitals, a Pastoral Care Department (PCD) oversees an agency wide plan to provide spiritual care for all clients. The program and policies of spiritual care developed by nurses need to be coordinated and complimentary to the efforts of the PCD. See Table 7, page 37, for an analysis of participation of many professional clergy and health care providers. This program functions in a multicultural, metropolitan area hospital near Washington D.C. in the USA, and it is necessarily very complex to meet the needs of the area. This is may serve as a sample for developing and coordinating nursing staff participation in spiritual care within your agency.

The support of agency board of trustee members and other administrators is an important facet to initiating and maintaining a program of spiritual care among nursing staff. Suggestions are offered in *An Administrator's Guide to Implementing Spiritual Care in Nursing Practice* (Battey, 2008).

Conclusion

There seems to be an innate pressure on humans to believe in something larger then themselves that has vast meaning for people. Through spirituality and religions, all of us seem to pose the following spiritual questions that we are trying our best to answer:

1. *Who are you?* What is your name? What is your true identity?
2. *Why are you here?* Why are you here in this particular place this day? But even more important: Why are you here on this planet at this time and place in history? What is your "calling"? What is your true reason for being? What is your true purpose for life?
3. *Where are you going?* In your life's journey, where are you headed? What do you seek to achieve? What is your true life's goal?
4. *Is there a life after death?* Is there a heaven? If there is, how do you get there? (Jones, 2001)

The point for nurses—for all of us—is this: give respect to the spiritual definitions, the beliefs, values, meanings, goals, and relationships that each person has chosen because, for that person, that definition is *the* right one. It would seem that, even with the ecumenical movement among religions, the Christians primarily, the continuing dialogues among the world's many religions, leaders will need to maintain their own beliefs and the identity of each religion. Too much history and culture is attached to each religion to merge into one universal belief system. (Smith, 1958, p.354-355) In the 21st century, we need to listen to our own chosen religion and remain true to our own beliefs. And we need to listen to the other religious beliefs as well as disbeliefs in order to understand them. We are living together on a planet that seems to grow smaller each day, given the ease of communication, travel, and exchange of knowledge, products—and illnesses. Nurses do become involved in personal lives and, for whatever theological or philosophical stance, these nurses need to show acceptance of the person, show compassion, and bring healing, wholeness, and peace.

This theory of spiritual care and accompanying educational and implementation suggestions are just that—suggestions. These ideas are offered, not as THE answer to the spiritual care issues, but as possibilities for consideration in your nursing practice and agency. Holistic health care is *the* paradigm of the 21st century. It's time to have a nursing theory of spiritual care to provide structure and direction in our practice. It's time, now.

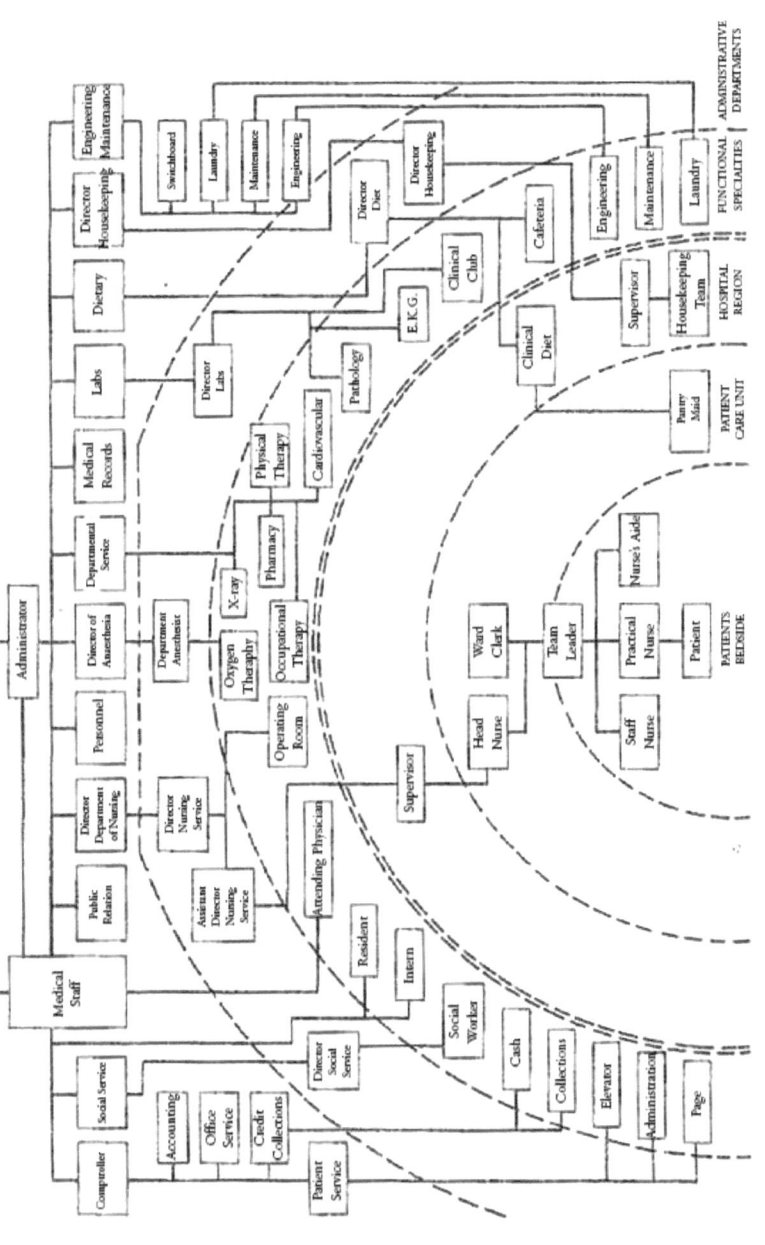

Figure 1 A half-circle hospital organizational chart, showing the patient as the central focus. The outward flow indicates the degree of functional and territorial social interaction hospital administrators and personnel have with the patient. (*From Mauksch, H.O. The nurse: Coordinator of patient care. In: J. K. Skipper, Jr., & R.C. Leonard, Social interaction and patient care. Philadelphia: Lippincott, 1965.*)

Figure 1. Half-Circle Organizational Chart

"This is a functional and territorial organization of a hospital, and the theme is client-centered care. The increasingly larger circles indicate the amount of contact, accountability, and responsibility the administrators, technicians, professionals, and others have with the patient. The chart conveys the power of the patient who is representative of society at large. It emphasizes a humanistic perspective of the client/patient as well as the need to satisfy each one by providing quality care, apparently the goal of the agency. It also clearly identifies who has the greatest opportunity and responsibility for speaking and acting as if a delegate for administrators—the clinical nurse. It presents the hospital as a nursing center where doctors practice occasionally and all other employees serve in a supportive capacity. Decades old, this model is seldom seen and rarely operationalized."[3]

---

[3]   Hersey, Paul & Duldt, Bonnie Weaver (Battey). (1989). *Situational Leadership in Nursing.* Norwalk, Conn.: Appleton-Lange, pp. 169-172.

Table 1. Assumptions

1) **Drawn from Existential Philosophy**.

   a) Existence predates essence (Sartre, 1973).
   b) A "reality" really exists "out there" and can be known through life experience; predestination is rejected (Claxton, 1984).
   c) Human beings are neither good nor evil, only that they develop "essence" through the choices made and actions taken (Vonnegut, 1969).
   d) Human beings are concerned with existential elements: being, becoming, choice, freedom, responsibility solitude, loneliness, pain, struggle, tragedy, meaning, dread, uncertainty despair, and death.
   e) The way things turn out provides sole "proof" or justification for whether an action was right or wrong (Vonnegut, 1969).
   f) Others are not to be blamed for the outcomes, but individuals assume full responsibility for one's own thoughts, feelings, and actions (Claxton, 1984; Burnard, 1989).
   g) Life experiences are interpreted by each individual so that a personal theory is developed, but it tends to differ from the "reality" out there (Claxton, 1984).
   h) Unable to escape from the "here and now," survival depends on the "communication imperative"; dialogue is necessary to share facts, feelings and coping strategies, especially when there is disagreement about "reality".

2) **Drawn from Theology**

   a) Spirituality is a part of human beings, an equal dimension with the body and mind, and it does not depend on religious/non-religious resources.
   b) The spirit is in charge of one's life, of the body and mind.
   c) Spirituality is a personal mystical experience.
   d) By tending to one's spiritual life, the health of one's body and mind tends to improve.

3) **Drawn from Nursing Practice**

   a) The purpose of nursing is to intervene to support, maintain, and augment the client's state of holistic health.

b) Human beings function as a unique, holistic (body, mind, and spirit) being responding openly to the environment.

c) All elements of existential beings are the salient issues to be dealt with in critical life situations by the communication imperative.

d) Interpersonal communication is a humanizing factor, an innate element of the nursing process occurring between nurses and clients, peers, and professional colleagues.

e) Evaluation of one's own communication skills is subjective; each person must make decisions and choices about communication behavior and choose to change, depending of ability to utilize feedback.

f) Humanizing communication can be learned, enhancing one's awareness and sensitivity to others (Battey, in press)

g) The goal is to break the communication cycle of dehumanizing attitudes and interaction patterns, replacing these with attitudes and patterns that humanize.

h) Nursing is existentialist in that it is practiced in the context of the moment in which opportunities to diagnose holistic discord and spiritual distress often occurs in multiple short, unplanned intervals.

i) In comparison with other health care providers, nurses are closest in proximity to the client on a 'round the clock basis.

Table 2 Concepts

1) **Holism:** Parts of any whole cannot exist and cannot be understood except in relation to the whole.

2) **Humans**: Holistic beings characterized by body (biophysical), mind (neurology and behavior) and spirit (soul, consciousness, energy fields.)

3) **Holistic Health**: A state in which the three integrated systems of body, mind and spirit function harmoniously as directed by the spirit.

4) **Holistic Discord and/or Spiritual Distress**: A *nursing diagnosis* based on human responses of anger, resentfulness, guilt, hopelessness, despair, depression, and a bland facial affect.

   a) **Related to:** being spiritually disconnected from the Creator, with significant relationships, with the goals and purposes for life, and even with awareness of one's own bodily signals of distress.

   b) **Evidenced by:** negative responses to life which includes a noncompliance to values, just "sticking it out," crying, whining and complaining, grieving over losses, and/or just no response at all . . . withdrawal into one's self. There is no peace. There is only discord.

5) **Spirituality:** A characteristic common to all human beings as expressed through attitudes; abstract and ethereal. (Battey, 2005, Lesson 8)

   a) **Religion:** A subset element of spirituality; a formal, organized practice within a faith community.

   b) **Client's Definition:** This definition is closely related to clients' health state and consists of a set of five elements: beliefs, values, meanings, goals, and relationships (BVMGR). The clients' spiritual care plan needs to focus on this personal definition, not a formal theological, religious, or philosophical definition.

      i) *Beliefs* that an "other" exists; that there is a universal force or power or energy that is creative and renewing. Who or what is my God or god(s). A continuum of "disbeliefs to neutral to beliefs."

      ii) *Values* or what is of ultimate importance in my life? How have I prioritized my resources? A continuum of negative to positive values.

iii) *Meanings* or what would I give up my life for? What are the significances or implications of my life's events, and what is happening to my body and mind?

iv) *Goals* or what is my "mission" in life? What am I called to do? What goals are appropriate? Where am I needed?

v) *Relationships* or what is the ultimate relationship or power in my life? What relationships do I need? What changes will occur as relationships are initiated, maintained, or ended, given what is happening to my body and mind? (Duldt & Pokorny, 1999; revised, Duldt-Battey, 2003, 2004).

6) **Spiritual Care:** Relational in nature through interpersonal communication (Kraus, in press).

a) The recipient (client) of spiritual care determines whether it exists at all.

b) Each existential individual has a personal definition of spirituality.

c) The nurse seeks to use the client's own definition of spirituality in developing an individualized plan of care.

7) **Nursing:** An academic discipline and practice profession concerned with the holistic care of people, healthy or ill, through prevention of illness, health maintenance, and health promotion across the life span.

a) **Elements of Nursing:**

i) **Communicating:** humanizing interpersonal communication.

ii) **Caring:** valuing, touching, and concern. A caring ambiance in the environment. (See Table 8, page 42 for suggested elements of caring.)

iii) **Coaching:** Teaching clients to care for ones' self to re-achieve, maintain health.

b) **Role of the Nurse in Spiritual Care:** to use humanizing communication as a positive influence on the client's spirit and to deliberately intervene with a high probability of success. (Battey, 2008)

i) **Recognize** the patient's distress and personal definition of spirituality using the rubric, BVMGR.

ii) **Respond** in a humanizing, compassionate manner.

    iii) **Record** according to ethical and legal guidelines and agency policies.

    iv) **Report** on a "need to know" basis to appropriate health care providers.

    v) **Refer** to appropriate spiritual advisor, such as a priest, rabbi, imam, or others. (Battey, 2008)

8) **Communication:** involves normal information-processing systems as one perceives, interprets, and responds to the environment. (See Humanizing Nursing Communication Theory, Battey, 2005, 2009).

    a) **Humanizing** means to make contact between people and build relationships.

    b) **Dehumanizing** means to break down interpersonal relationships and lose contact.

9) **Health:** An individual's state of being, of becoming, or self-awareness. An existential, free flowing state in one's particular spot in the time/space/relationship intersection.

10) **Critical Life Situations:** Involves the perception that one's existential state of being is in jeopardy, as in the event of illness, accidents, and/or dying.

    a) Changes in health/illness state may be necessary to cope with critical life situation.

    b) Interaction of all characteristics of being human increases in trying to cope (see assumption #1-d, page 18).

11) **Environment:** One's time/space/relationship context which provides each individual a unique "frame of reference." It includes all physical and social interactions.

12) **Allostasis**, Meaning "maintaining stability (homeostasis) through change" (Sterling and Eyer, 1988; McEwen, 1998, 1999a).

    a) **Allostasis load:** Refers to the wear and tear one's body experiences from going through many cycles of allostasis stress responses, repeatedly turning the system on and off.

    b) **Allostasis load disorders**: The range of illnesses associated with the dysfunction of the allostatic system.

13) **Ten "markers" of spiritual distress:** Allostatic load disorders from spiritual distress are associated with positive physical markers which are predictors of disease and deterioration of the human system.

    a) The 10 "markers": 12 hour overnight excretions of 1) cortisone, 2) nor-epinephrine, 3) epinephrine, 4) serum DHEAS levels; also 5) average systolic BP, 6) average diastolic BP, 7) waist to hip circumference ratio, 8) serum HDL, 9) cholesterol to HDL ratio, and 10) Hemoglobin A1C level. (Fricchione, 2004).

    b) These markers can serve as a guide for recognizing spiritual distress.

14) **Stress Buffering:** Interventions to reduce stress and increase the probability of resilience and ultimate healing.

    a) **Cognitive Behavioral Therapy**: Teaching the client to substitute positive thoughts for negative ones.

    b) **Relaxation Response**: Using prayer or meditation to focus and relax (Benson, 1975).

    c) **Social Support**: A warm, accepting social climate.

    d) **Complimentary and Alternative Therapies**: The multidimensional model of healing energies such as acupuncture, therapeutic touch and distance healing as well as crystals, herbal remedies, homeopathic medicine, Yoga, Reiki, Q Gong, color and light therapies, and music therapy to name a few.

15) **Resiliency:** The capability to withstand stress (Fricchione, 2004).

    a) Continuing to be *optimistic* during stressful situations.

    b) Learned *helpfulness*; responding with *effective behaviors* in spite of fear.

    c) Maintaining *social bonding*, team work, and a sense of selflessness or altruism.

Table 3. Relationship Statements

1) Holistic health equals the product of the sum of the mind times the body times the spirit times the environment.

a) Holistic Health = Environment (Mind x Body x Spirit) (Battey & Acree, 2007)
b) ↑Holistic Health = ↑ Resiliency

2) If stress buffering interventions are applied, then there is a high probability that allostatic loading and spiritual distress will decrease, so that resilience is increased, leading to a greater degree of holistic health for the client.

   a) Stress Buffering Interventions → ↓ allostatic loading → ↓ spiritual distress = ↑ Resilience → ↑ Holistic Health

      i) Cognitive Behavioral Therapy intervention = ↑ Resilience
      ii) Relaxation Response intervention = ↑ Resilience
      iii) Social Support intervention = ↑ Resilience
      iv) Complimentary and Alternative Therapies interventions = ↑ Resilience

3) If one uses humanizing nursing communication and ethics theories in creating an ambiance of *caring* in the patient's environment, then there is a high probability that social support will be increased, allostatic loading decreased, and spiritual distress decreased so that resilience is increased, leading achieving a greater degree holistic health for the patient/client.

   a) If HNCT + HNCET + Caring of Nurse = ↑ Social Support
   b) (Mind x Body x Spirit) x (Stress Buffering x Caring) =↑ Resilience
   c) CBT + RR + SS+ C/A x (B x M x S) = ↑ Residency

Table 4. Evaluation

1) **Relevant research.**

    a) Extensive research programs are clustered around centers in the United States such as the following, plus many others:

        i) The Benson-Henry Institute of the Massachusetts General Hospital in Boston;

        ii) The Center of Spirituality, Theology, and Health at Duke University in Durham, North Carolina

        iii) The George Washington University Institute for Spirituality and Health in Washington, D. C.

        iv) The Faith and Health Connection in Charlotte, North Carolina.

    b) Extensive research funding resources are also clustered about the concepts of "mind-body connection", "spirituality and health" through the National Institute of Health in Washington D.C.

    c) Studies about spirituality are also conducted at research centers located in numerous universities such as the University of Minnesota, Harvard University, and the University of California at San Francisco and at Los Angeles as well.

2) **Importance to the discipline and profession.**

    a) This theory defines a limited scope of practice of spiritual care for professional nurses.

    b) The scope is confined to the contexts in which nurses commonly practice as opposed to the extensive contexts of chaplains, priests, rabbi, or other clergy.

3) **Parsimony.**

    a) The theory of spirituality is organized into consecutive elements which are listed in subsets. The assumptions, concepts and relationship statements are grouped for clarity and ease of identification.

b) The concepts' definitions are clearly and concisely defined to apply to multiple contexts and beliefs regarding spirituality and religion.

c) The relationship statements follow logical or principle formats to foster application to research hypotheses and questions as well as statistical analysis.

4) **Scope.**

a) The theory of spirituality is designed to apply to all general and specialty areas of nursing practice.

b) The theory limits the scope of spiritual care for nursing for the novice or those who reject spirituality; it does provide a reasonable basis for incorporating spiritual care by nurses holding any view of spirituality and its subset, religion.

c) The theory allows an expanded practice for those individual nurses who are caring for clients of their own faith community or who choose to do more in selected cases.

5) **Limitations.**

a) To include spiritual and religious practices, such as prayer or baptism, all nurses are ethically and legally responsible for obtaining the client's (or families') consent.

6) **Applicability.**

a) It is particularly appropriate for introductory courses in nursing education as well as practice specialties such as oncology and hospice.

b) It is designed to meet minimal criteria and standards for accreditation and professional codes of ethics.

7) **Generalizability and agreement with known data.**

a) The assessment (10 markers) and four interventions are based on recent findings of medical research.

b) Support of the Nursing Theory of Spiritual Care is provided by numerous research studies conducted in a wide range of public health and health care professions as well as theological and religious investigators.

Table 5. Spiritual Care Map.[4]

Beliefs	Values	Meanings

Goals	Client/Patient'sName: Age: Other: Health Status:	Relationships

Nursing Diagnosis *Spiritual Distress related to:* *As evidenced by:* *Objective:* *Subjective:* *Intervention:*	Recording: Reporting: Referring:

4 Battey, B W. (2005). *Faith community (parish) nursing: A computer assisted instruction (CAI) program*. (Note: All CAI programs are available from *http://www.askdatasystems.com./*)

Table 6

Cancer Case[5]	Clustering Evidence:
Patient: Female, 30 years old admitted through ER, sent to ICU overnight; transferred to Medical unit for continued observation.	**Nursing Diagnosis:** Spiritual distress related to:
Diagnosis: Acute abdominal pain; ovarian cancer, Stage IV.	**As evidenced by:** Objective:
Prognosis: Poor. Estimated 6 months to live. Refer to Hospice.	Subjective:
Communication: As nurse gives morning care, medications, etc., she states: "I have three small children, and I won't be able to have an influence on their growing up. I won't be there for their graduations, marriages, or births of my grandchildren. There are so many thing I expected to be able to say to them."	**Responding; Intervention:** **Recording:** **Reporting:**
Focus: 1. Ethical Issues 2. Other:	**Referring:**

5   Battey, B W. (2005). *Faith community (parish) nursing: A computer assisted instruction (CAI) program.* (Available from *http://www.askdatasystems.com./*)

Table 7. Services and activities of an ecumenical hospital Pastoral Care Departments (PCD) which may be incorporated into the practices of a variety of health care professionals' practice and members of local community.[6]

Services and Activities of Pastoral Care Departments (PCD)	Professional Ministry: Clergy, Rabbi, Priests, Diaconal Ministers and Deaconesses.	Pastoral Care Department Volunteer Lay Chaplains	Doctors, Nurses, Psychiatrists, Physical Therapists, and similar health care professionals	Community Clergy, Parish Nurses, Sisters, Brothers, and Faith Community.
1. Conduct formal services	Yes			Yes
2. Serve Communion	Yes			Yes
3. Baptize	Yes	Yes	Yes	Yes
4. Classic Healing Service: Anointing with oil and laying on of hands	Yes In Chapel and at bedside	Yes At bedside	Yes At bedside	Yes At bedside, at health care agency, and/or home.
5. Ethics Committee Screening	Yes Chaplain convener of committee; others may also be members.	Yes Referrals	Yes Referrals, member	Yes Referrals
6. Visit, pray with patients, families	Yes	Yes Regular Duty	Yes	Yes
7. Rounds; on call 24 hr. daily for spiritual needs.	Yes Chaplains administrative assignment	Yes Regular duty	Yes Referrals to Pastoral Care Department	Yes Visit members of own faith community per request
8. Blessing and Naming Ceremony for Stillborn	Yes	Yes Regular duty, but voluntary	Yes Witness, participation optional	Yes Witness, participation optional
9. Educational Programs for PCD	Yes Chaplains administratively assignment	Yes	Yes	Yes
10. Conduct Ecumenical Hospital Services	Yes Chaplains Regular Duty	Yes Optional	Yes May volunteer	Yes Optional
11. Conduct support groups for cancer, other patient and/or family groups	Yes Administratively authorizes	Yes Optional		Yes Optional

[6]   Duldt, B. W. The spiritual dimension of holistic care. (2002). *Journal of Nursing Administration*, 32(1), 20-24. Revised, B.W. Battey, March, 2009.

12. Special Role Educational criteria	Yes Clinical Pastoral Education (CPE) by Certified Clinical Chaplain	Yes Orientation to Lay Chaplaincy required; recommendation by an ecclesiastical body, a college degree, and course on pastoral care	Yes May volunteer to help in teaching orientation and courses on pastoral care	Yes As required or assigned
13. Orientation to Lay Chaplain role in ER, Psyc. Unit and other specialty units.		Yes Voluntary assignment		
14. Mentor to Seminary Intern and Resident Chaplains	Yes Regular Duty	Yes Assigned mentoring, voluntary		Yes
15. Remain with critically ill patient, family	Yes	Yes Regular Duty	(No time for this)	Yes Optional
16. Respond to Code Blue; stay with family, patient roommate	Yes	Yes Regular duty, comfort family, roommate, liaison to nurses and doctors.	(No time – need to focus on code)	(Probably not available)
17. Remain with family after death.	Yes	Yes Regular Duty	(No time for this)	Yes
18. Take family to morgue, etc.	Yes Per hospital policy	Yes Regular duty per hospital policy	Yes By policy, unit personnel accompany family	Yes May be invited if available.
19. Visit, pray and give blessing to premature infants, parents.	Yes	Yes Regular duty		Yes Optional
20. Visit patients hospitalized over 5 days.	Yes	Yes Regular duty		Yes
21. Listen to patient/family concerns, serve as	Yes	Yes	Yes	Yes

advocate, liaison, etc.				
22. Maintain supply of communion sets, oil, baptismal shell, candles, Bibles, etc.	Yes	Yes		
23. Report deaths to Regional Organ Transplant agency	Yes Administrative assignment	Yes Regular duty per hospital policy		
24. Provide information about Organ Donations, Living Wills and other end of life issues.	Yes	Yes	Yes	Yes
25. Maintain records of visits, interventions, and reactions; maintain confidentiality.	Yes	Yes Regular duty to log activities	Yes	Yes
26. Serve on Pastoral Care Committee: set policy, evaluate, implement, and support DPC	Yes		Yes Usually dctors, nurses, administrators, patients and community clergy.	
27. Public presentations to community groups regarding PCD per request, assignment	Yes	Yes	Yes	Yes

Table 8. Elements of Caring[7]

In the book, Sweitzer, David K. *Pastoral Care Emergencies: Ministering to People in Crisis* (Minneapolis: Fortress Press, 2000). Switzer addresses brief care for people who are experiencing personal and family emergencies. On pages 12 & 13 he quotes Mayeroff's list of "Ingredients of caring" which could be applicable to nurses:

1) Knowledge: an understanding of the other person's needs and the competency to respond to them.
2) The capacity for self-evaluation: the ability to look critically at our own behavior in relationship to the other person.
3) Patience: staying with the person as she/he is enabled to grow at her/his own time and space.
4) Trust: trust in process, the relationship, the other person's possibilities and trust in the Holy Spirit.
5) Honesty: seeing oneself and the other as we actually are and not as we would like to present ourselves.
6) Humility: never allowing ourselves to think that we know all there is to know about the other person or ourselves—the recognition of our limitations.
7) Hope: in regard to what will happen to and for the other person as a result of our caring.
8) Courage: a necessary prerequisite for the hope just described. There is a risk involved in investing ourselves as we do in any caring for another without knowing the outcome. Courage is going into the unknown with another.

---

[7]   Schmalenberger, J. (Personal Communication, March 26, 2009.)

References

Aiken, L., Smith, H., and Lake, E. (1994). Lower Medicare mortality among a set of hospital known for good nursing care. *Medical Care*, 32(8), 771-787.

Aiken L. H., et al. (2001). Nurses' reports on hospital care in five countries. *Health Affairs*. 20(3):43-53, May-June.

_____ *ANA Agenda for Health Care Reform*. Washington D.C.: American Nurses Publishing. Downloaded June 28, 2005.

American Nurses' Association. (2003). *Nursing's social policy statement*, 2nd ed., Washington, DC. *http://www.nursesbooks.org*

American Nurses Association. (2001). *Code of ethics for nurses with interpretive statements*. Washington, DC: American Nurses Publishing.

Barnum, B. S. (2003). *Spirituality in Nursing: From traditional to new age.* 2nd. ed. New York: Springer Publishing Company.

Battey. B. W. (in press). *Spirituality in nursing practice: A computer assisted instructional program.* Companion booklet: Course Manual. (Note: All CAI programs are available from http://www.askdatasystems.com./)

Battey, B. W. (2008). *Administrator's guide to implementing spiritual care into nursing practice.* Philadelphia: Xlibris Corporation. *www.Order. Xlibris.com.*

Battey, B. W. (2005). Humanizing Nursing Communication Theory. (An analysis is available for downloading from the website: *http://www. bwbatteyconsult.com*)

Battey, B. W. & Acree, J.R. (2006). Spiritual Assessment in Health Care: Guidelines for providing the Third Dimension of Holistic Health Care: Participant's Manual. (A workshop for staff nursing and other health care providers.) Antioch, Ca.

Battey, B W. (2005). *Faith community (parish) nursing: A computer assisted instruction (CAI) program.* (Note: All CAI programs are available from *http://www.askdatasystems.com./*)

Beckman, L. F., & S. L. Syme. (1979) Social network, host resistance, and mortality: A nine year follow-up study of Alameda County residents. *American Journal of Epidemiology.* 109" 186-204.

Benson, H. (1975). *The relaxation response.* New York: Avon.

Benson, Herbert. (2004). The power of belief and the role of relaxation in health care. *Spirituality and healing in medicine: The enhanced importance of the integration of mind/body practices and prayer.* (A continuing education course sponsored by the Harvard Medical, the Mind/Body Medical Institute, and George Washington University, and the George Washington Institute for Spirituality and Health.) Boston: December 11-12, 2004.

Benson, Herbert, and William Proctor. (2003). *Break-Out Principle.* New York: Scribner.

Berman, A., Snyder, S. J., Lozier, B., & Erb, G. (2007). *Kozier & Erb's fundamentals of nursing: Concepts, process, and practice.* 8th Ed. Upper Saddle River, N.J.: Prentice Hall Health.

Buber, M. (1970). *I and Thou.* Translated by Walter Kaufmann. New York: Charles Scribner's Sons.

Buerhaus, Peter I. (2005). Six-Part series on the State of the RN workforce in the United States. *Nursing Economics,* 23(2), 58-69.

Buerhaus, P., Donelan, K., Ulrich, B., Des Roches, C., Normal, L., and Dittus, R. (2007). Impact of the nurse shortage on hospital patient care: Comparative perspectives. *Health Affairs,* 26(3), 853-62.

Buerhaus, P., et al. (2007). Trends in the experiences of hospital-employed registered nurses: Results from three national survey. *Nursing Economics.* 25(2);69-80.

Buerhaus, P., Donelan, K., Norman, L., & Dittus, R. (2005). Nursing student's perceptions of a career in nursing and impact of a national campaign designed to attract people into the nursing profession. *Journal of Professional Nursing,* 21(2):75-83

Burnard, P. (1989). Existentialism as a theoretical basis for counseling in psychiatric nursing. *Archives of Psychiatric Nursing,* 3, 142-147.

Carson, V.S. (2000). *Mental health nursing: The nurse-patient journey.* 2nd Ed. Philadelphia: Saunders.

Carson, V. S. and Koenig, H. G. (2004) *Spiritual caregiving; Health care as a ministry.* Philadelphia and London: Templeton Foundation Press.

Claxton, G. (1984). *Live and learn: An introduction to the psychology of growth and change in everyday life.* London: Harper & Row.

Dossey, Larry. (1993). *Healing Words: The Power of Prayer and the Practice of Medicine.* New York: Harper Collins.

Duldt, B. W. & Pokorny, M. (1999) Teaching Communication about Human Sexuality to Nurses and other Health Care Providers. *Nurse Educator,* 24(5),27-32.

Duldt (Battey), B.W. & K. Giffin. (1985). *Theoretical Perspectives for Nursing.* Boston: Little Brown & Company.

Enright, R.D. (2001). *Forgiveness is a choice: A step-by-step process for resolving anger and restoring hope.* Washington, D. C.: American Psychological Association.

Flanigan, Beverly. (1992). *Forgiving the unforgivable: Overcoming the bitter legacy of intimate wounds.* New York: Wiley Publishing, Inc.

Fricchione, Gregory L. (2004). The potential for illness prevention via spirit-mind-body approaches. *Spirituality and healing in medicine: The enhanced importance of the integration of mind/body practices and prayer.* (A continuing education course sponsored by the Harvard Medical, the Mind/Body Medical Institute, and George Washington University, and the George Washington Institute for Spirituality and Health.) Boston: December 11-12, 2004.

Hersey, P. & B.W. (Battey) Duldt. (1985). *Situational Leadership in Nursing.* East Norwalk, Conn.: Appleton-Lange.

Hitchcock, J.E., Schubert, P.E., & Thomas, S.H. (2003). *Community health nursing: Caring in action.* Albany, N.Y.: Delmar.

Holmes, Thomas, & Richard Rahe (1967). Holmes-Rahe life changes scale. *Journal of Psychosomatic Research,* Vol. 11, pp. 213-218. To view the scale, go to (retrieved September, 28, 2008): *http://www.geocities.com/beyond_stretched/holmes.htm http://www.markhenri.com/health/stress.html*

Joint Commission on Accreditation of Healthcare Organizations. (Retrieved April 7, 2009) *http://www.jointcommission.org/, http://www.jcrinc.com/Search/spiritual* and *http://www.jcrinc.com/Organizational-Ethics-Statements/Ethics-Committee/Organizational-Ethics-Issues/*

Jones, Robert, The Rev., Pastor. (June 24, 2001) Sermon: "Who are we, Why are we here? Where are we going?" Front Royal, VA: Good Shepherd Evangelical Lutheran Church.

Koenig, H. G. (2002). *Spirituality in patient care: Why, how, when, and what.* Philadelphia & London: Templeton Press.

Kraus, Paul. (in press). Pastoral care: A computer assisted instruction for nursing and allied health. (Note: CAI programs are available from *http:// www.askdatasystems.com./*)

Leininger M. (1978). *Transcultural nursing: Concepts, theories and practices.* New York, NY: Wiley.

Lemmer, C. (2002). Teaching the spiritual dimension of nursing care: A survey of U.S. Baccalaureate nursing programs. *Journal of Nursing Education*, 41(11): 482-490.

Levin, Jeff. (2001). *God, faith, and health: Exploring the spirituality-healing connection.* New York: John Wiley & Sons, Inc.

O'Brien, M. E. (1999). *Spirituality in nursing: Standing on holy ground.* Sudbury, MA: Jones and Bartlett.

Macrae, J. (1995). Nightingale's spiritual philosophy and its significance for modern nursing. *Image: Journal of Nursing Scholarship*, 27, 8-10.

McEwen, M. (2004). Analysis of spirituality content in nursing textbooks. *Journal of Nursing Education*, 43(1):20-30.

McEwen, B. S. (1998). Protective and damaging effects of stress mediators. *New England Journal of Medicine*, 338: 171-179.

McEwen, B. S. & Seaman, T. (1999). Protective and damaging effects of mediators or stress: Elaborating and testing the concepts of allostasis and allostatic load. *Annuals of New York Academy of Science*, 896:30-37.

McEwen, B. & Krahn, D. (1999). The response to stress. *The Doctor Will See You Now. http://www.thedoctorwillseeyounow.com/articles/behavior/ stress_3/index.shtml*

McSherry, W. (2006). *Making sense of spirituality in nursing and health care practice: An interactive approach.* 2nd Ed. London & Philadelphia: Jessica Kingsley Publishers.

McSherry, W., & Cash, K. (2004). The language of spirituality: an emerging taxonomy. *International Journal of Nursing Studies* 41: 1511-161.

McSherry, & W, L Ross. (2002). Dilemmas of spiritual assessment: Considerations for nursing practice. *Journal of Advanced Nursing.* 38(5): 479-88.

Matthews, Dale A., M.D. (1999). *The faith factor: proof of the healing power of prayer.* New York: Penguin Books.

Meyer, C.L. (2003). How effectively are nurse educators preparing students to provide spiritual care? *Nurse Educator*, 28:185-90.

National Institute for Health and Clinical Excellence. (2006). *Depression and anxiety—computerised cognitive behavioural therapy Retrieved August 15, 2007: http://www.nice.org.uk/guidance/TA97*

Nielsen L, Seaman T, & Hahn A. (2007). *NIA Exploratory Workshop on Allostatic Load.* Washington, DC: Behavioral and Social Research Program, *National Institute on Aging, and National Institutes of Health. www.nia. nih.gov/ . . . /AF0997F6-0C16-4A76-96C0-D3780F00E6D4/8839/ AllostaticLoadBackgroundMaterials.doc—02-28-2009* (Retrived March, 2009)

Neuman, B. (1982a). *The Neuman systems model: Applications to nursing education and practice.* Norwalk, Connecticut: Appleton Lange.

Nichols, W. R., (Ed.) (1999). *Random House Webster's College Dictionary.* New York: Random House.

Nightingale, F. (1959). *Notes on Nursing: What it is, and what it is not.* 5th Ed. London: Harrison, 59, Pall Mall, 1959. A facsimile reproduced from the copy in the Rare Book Room from the Library of Congress, Washington D.C., Published by J. B. Lippincott Company, Philadelphia, 1946.

Nightingale, Florence. (1859). *Notes on Nursing.* London: Harrison, 59, Pall Mall, Bookseller to the Queen. Reprinted, 1946: Philadelphia: Edward Stern & Company, Inc.

North American Nursing Diagnosis Association. (2008) *Nursing diagnoses: definitions and classification, 2003-2004.* Philadelphia: Nanda International, pp. 208-209.

Patterson, J. & L. Zderad. (1976). *Humanistic Nursing.* New York: John Wiley Sons, Inc.

Selye, H. (1973). The evolution of the stress concept. *American Science,* 61:692-699.

Schmalenberger, J. (Personal communication, March 31, 2009).

Sartre, Jean-Paul. (1957). *Existentialism and humanism.* Translated and with an introduction by Philip Mairet. Brooklyn: Hastings House.

Shea, J. (2000). *Spirituality & health care: Reaching toward a holistic future.* Chicago: The Park Ridge Center for the Study of Health, Faith, and Ethics.

Smith, Huston. (1958). *The religions of man.* New York: Harper & Row, Publishers.

Sterling, P. & J. Eyer. (1988). Allostasis: A new paradigm to explain arousal pathology. In: Fisher, S., Reason J., editors. *Handbook of life stress, cognition and health.* New York: John Wiley and Sons.

Sweitzer, D. K. (2000). *Pastoral Care Emergencies: Ministering to People in Crisis.* Minneapolis: Fortress Press.

Taylor, El J. (2002). *Spiritual Care: Nursing theory, research, and practice.* Upper Saddle River, New Jersey: Prentice Hall.

Vonnegut, K. (1969). *Mother night.* London: Cape.

Other Sites and References of Interest

The Society for Spirituality, Theology & Health; Box 3825; Duke University Medical Center; Durham, North Carolina 27710. *http://www.societysth. org/*

American Holistic Nurses Association; 323 N. San Francisco Street, Suite 201

Flagstaff, AZ 86001. *http://www.ahna.org/*

Membership of Religions. *http://religion-cults.com/Overview/MEMBERSHIP. htm*

Battey, B. W. (2004). Chapter 8: Communication, Persuasion, and Negotiation. In: Diane Huber, (ed.), *Leadership and Nursing Care Management*, 4th Edition. St. Louis: ELSEVIER Mosby: Saunders.

Duldt-Battey, B. W. (2004). Using the holistic paradigm in teaching. In: Oermann, M. H., editor, *Annual Review of Nursing Education*, Vol. 2. New York: Springer Publishing Company.

Duldt (Battey), B. W. (2002). The spiritual dimension of holistic care. Journal of Nursing Administration, 32:1, pp. 20-24.

Duldt (Battey) B. W. (2001) Anatomy of a theory: A computer assisted instructional (CAI) program; Instructor's manual and Student workbook. (Note: CAI programs are available from *http://www.askdatasystems. com./*)

Duldt (Battey), B. W. (1991). "I-Thou": Research supporting humanistic nursing communication theory. *Perspectives of Psychiatric Care*, 27(3), 5-12.

Author's Biography

Bonnie Weaver Battey, Ph.D., R.N., is a nursing consultant in private practice, serving nursing education clients nationally and internationally. She completed her undergraduate work at Valparaiso University and Wagner College, receiving a BS degree in Nursing, and she received a MSN in Nursing Education degree from Vanderbilt University. She completed a thesis research survey on "Patients' Opinions on Visitors." She earned her Ph.D. at the University of Kansas, Lawrence, majoring in Speech Communication and Human Relations. Her dissertation was titled "Anger, Cohesiveness, and Productivity in Small Task Groups." She was a recipient of the Nurse Scientist Scholar grant for her doctoral studies. Post doctoral work included the Advanced Quantitative Methodology Institute, National Center for Nursing Research, St. Mary's Maryland, July 25-31, 1992. She was one of 60 nurse faculty/researchers selected nationally. Dr. Battey is listed in Who's Who among American Nurses," 1988-1995, "Who's Who in American Education." 2007-2008, "Who's Who in America," 2009, and "2000 Outstanding Intellectuals of the 21st Century."

As a tenured professor at East Carolina University, Dr. Battey has taught all levels of Medical Surgical or Adult Health clinical nursing courses, from introductory courses and health assessment skills laboratories to advanced clinical courses. She has also taught nursing leadership, theories, research, education, curriculum development, death and dying, as well as interdisciplinary speech, and ethics/philosophy courses. She has supervised the research of numerous graduate students' thesis, and conducted her own research in nursing communication to investigate her theory of Humanizing Nursing Communication and Ethics. She has also served as adjunct faculty at George Mason University as well as several other universities.

In addition to serving as faculty, Dr. Battey has served as administrator of associate degree, baccalaureate, and master's programs in nursing, and initiated an ADN and a BSN program in nursing. She served as an accreditation visitor over 25 years for undergraduate and graduate levels of nursing education programs. Dr. Battey has authored numerous articles, chapters, and several books as well as given presentations at professional and lay conferences and meetings on a variety of issues about nursing and research. She has also authored four computer assisted instruction programs for distance education. She has served on numerous committees for state boards of nursing and nursing associations, and she is a member of Sigma Theta Tau International and the Society for Spirituality, Theology and Health, The American Holistic Nurses' Association, and the Health Ministries Association.

Volunteer community services have included eight years as Parish Nurse at Good Shepherd Lutheran Church, Front Royal, Virginia and Nativity Evangelical Lutheran Church, Alexandria, Virginia. She has also served on numerous boards, such as the steering committee for establishing St. Luke (free) Community Clinic, Front Royal, Virginia.

Dr. Battey also served for four years as a Lay chaplain in Chaplaincy Program of INOVA Alexandria Hospital, Alexandria, Virginia. Her two primary mentors included the Director of Pastoral Care, Chaplain J. Vincent Guss Jr., D.Min(c), an ordained Lutheran minister, and a Board Certified Chaplain through the Association of Professional Chaplains; and Kathy A. Garrison, MAR, Director, Art of Pastoral Care, Pastoral Counseling of Northern Virginia, a Lutheran Deaconess, and a Diaconal Minister of the ELCA.